Working from Home

Mastering the Art of Sitting at Your Computer

Dr. Mitchell A. Kershner, N.D.

Naturopathic Doctor

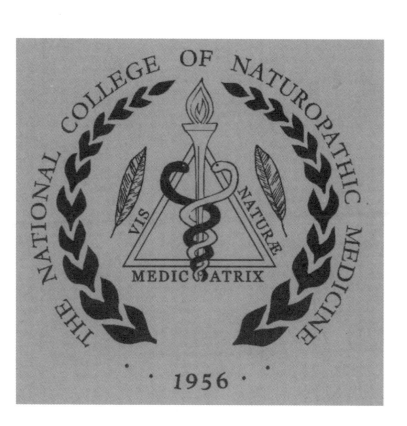

THE NATIONAL COLLEGE OF NATUROPATHIC MEDICINE

VIS NATURÆ MEDICATRIX

· 1956 ·

DEDICATION

I would like to dedicate this book to three very important people in my life who have been tremendously supportive. First is my mom Sherry; many would refer to her as a stepmother, but for me, she's a second mom. Second is my aunt Elinor, with whom I have gotten to share many a thought and idea; she is always there as a sounding board with her straightforward opinions. And last, my dearly departed grandmother Dora, whom we referred to as Nana growing up. Dora saw in me what no one else seemed to recognize that I could do anything I chose to put my mind and abilities to. She instilled a faith and belief that has stayed with me these last thirty years.

ACKNOWLEDGMENT

I have heard that Mahatma Gandhi once said, "It takes a village to raise a child." The same holds true for writing and sharing one's message. This work is being brought to all those in need of staying healthy at their computer and other devices. Gratitude also goes to all the patients I saw during my practice days. They inspired me with their stories of making the changes we discussed, proving what a difference a few preventative measures can make in their well-being.

Thanks to all my family members who understood when I couldn't show up for family affairs and for all the support they offered. I especially thank my sister, who does not always understand what I'm doing but always supports my efforts. Lastly, thanks to all of you who are willing to incorporate these tips and techniques in an attempt to prevent computer-related injuries (CRI) from affecting your quality of life.

CONTENTS

INTRODUCTION

How many times have you looked up from the computer and wondered where the time went? Computers, tablets, smartphones—whatever the form—these devices are consuming more of our time and thus affecting our overall health. From neck and back pain to joint stiffness, eye strain, irritability, and trouble sleeping, your favorite little toy is taking a toll on your health. But it doesn't have to. We no longer "look up" information—we Google it. We connect with anyone, anywhere, anytime. We use software programs and apps to simplify our lives and relieve some of our mental burdens. And we do this—on average—eight hours a day, every day, according to Kelton research. Demographics in America show our youth are plugging into their computers more and watching television less, according to the 2011 Youth Risk Behavior Surveillance Survey released by the Centers for Disease Control and Prevention (CDC). Who knew it would come with such a cost to our bodies and minds?

Although computer-related injuries are mostly physical, there is a mental component. As strange as it may sound, I sometimes have to push myself to leave my home office for things like going to the gym, even though working out is an integral part of my life. As a naturopath, I know better—yet it still happens. The workplace scene has undergone dramatic changes. Many more people today are setting up "shop"—offices in their own homes. Although this has advantages, such as cost savings on office space and other expenses, there are disadvantages to staying at home. Lack of in-person workplace interaction can lead to loneliness, which can lead to mild or moderate depression. As a result, there is an uncategorized condition known as Social Media Depression.

Although not listed in the *Diagnostic and Statistical Manual of Mental Disorders* (known as the DSM), this condition is becoming more recognized because of isolation with home computer use. Excessive media use, in general, can lead to depression, particularly among teenagers.

The list of physical conditions related to improper overuse of devices is long, from the familiar such as Carpal Tunnel Syndrome, migraines, joint stiffness, and low back pain, to catch-all terms such as work-related upper limb disorder and musculoskeletal disorder. Medical professionals group all these ailments under the umbrella term computer-related injuries. The injuries involve many systems of the body and can occur at any age. No computer users, including children, are immune. The following is a list of common computer-related injuries:

- Carpal Tunnel Syndrome
- Migraines
- Computer Vision Syndrome

- Occupational Overuse Syndrome
- Joint Stiffness
- Low Back Pain

Here's the hard truth about these injuries: they're not the fault of the devices. It's all operator error. We are so engrossed in catching up on Facebook or playing games or working that we rarely move anything except our fingers from the time we log on until when we log off. And we strategically place all the necessary computer-related components—ink, printer, fax, and phone—nearby. I even have the remote for the radio on my office desk so I don't have to get up to change the station. A friend of mine has a mini refrigerator under her desk so snacks and drinks are within reach.

For years, my patients have struggled to overcome computer-related injuries. For them, and for you, I have a saying: "Where there is a problem or challenge, there is a solution. It's a matter of finding it." This book contains some simple, yet effective, strategies to combat computer-related injuries—simple means, methods, and cost-effective ways to stay healthy while at your computer. Read on to learn how to find balance by applying principles that can help you prevent Computer-Related Injuries (CRIs) from your long-term use of computers. This is what the "Simple Solution" in each chapter is devoted to. These tips come from my years in private practice discerning treatments that have worked with my patients. My hope is that they will work for you and lessen any need for further treatments. By preventing today, there won't be a need to treat tomorrow.

1

Setting the Tone of Your Day

WHEN ORANGE JUICE JUST ISN'T ENOUGH

The definition of breakfast is literally breaking a fast. Typically, when you wake up, you've gone ten to twelve hours without eating or drinking anything. And if you are like most people, your morning routine is filled with getting ready to meet the day in as organized a manner as possible. Running around gathering your papers, keys, or whatever you're going to need for the day, there usually isn't much time for eating. Coffee machines handle the brewing process so you can fill a to-go cup as you head out the door.

There are better ways to prepare your body and brain for the day ahead.

During a good night's sleep, the heart continues to beat, albeit slower usually. Breathing, digesting, making hormones, and dreaming are all going on. Body temperature is maintained throughout the night. This is why we have a strong tendency to be in a state of dehydration first thing in the morning.

By drinking a strong caffeine drink such as coffee or a sugary drink like soda, the adrenal glands are shocked into action and the pancreas is forced to start the flow of insulin in high quantities. Both types of liquids start your day with blood sugar spikes and put a strain on brain function. This will have an adverse effect on how the rest of your day will go. Mood swings, poor concentration, energy drop in the afternoon, and many other symptoms are associated with stimulating your adrenals like this first thing in the morning. Artificial sweeteners do not appear to be any better. Relatively recent research has produced evidence to support that they, too, have a poor reaction with spiking blood sugar levels. At this time, it would be best to avoid artificial sweeteners as we don't know enough about how they affect long-term brain activity.

After years of patient contacts and thousands of medical history intakes, I have learned that how individuals start their day usually dictates how their day will shape up. I make it a point to begin my day by drinking a glass of water; just because I have been relatively inactive, that doesn't mean my body was on hold.

Tight Neck and Shoulders

Many people complain of tightness in the neck and shoulders as their days wear on. Posture is a crucial feature to prevent decreased range of motion. If sitting for many hours is how you're going to spend your day, you would benefit from a good stretch or yoga routine in the morning. Stretching and yoga, in my opinion, are the most important form of exercise.

Since tendons and ligaments are responsible for holding our bones and muscles together, it's important to keep them supple and flexible. As we age, our tendons and ligaments tend to shorten from lack of stretching. When this happens, people can add reduced joint flexibility and shortened muscle length to common complaints of physical aches and pains. It is one thing to have strong muscles, but it's more important to be flexible and have a greater range of movement as we age. When patients tell me how getting up in the morning is becoming more challenging, one of my recommendations is to start the day with an easy stretching routine.

It is usually a good idea to take a class to learn proper techniques, in hopes of preventing any injuries, and the rewards of a more flexible body will be worth every achy stretch move. There is usually an initial learning curve and physical adjustment, but after a few weeks and months, not stretching will be missed by the body. I start just about every day with stretching or yoga, and afterward, I make a cup of herbal tea or hot lemon water with a touch of honey.

In a stretching routine or some form of exercise, I include meditation and prayer. This time allows for getting focused on what is most important and helps define why I'm going to do what I've set my goals on for the day. During this time, there is reflection on gratitude for all the wonderful things in life, such as good food, access to clean water, and freedom to pursue my dreams. After completing meditation and first morning liquids, I eat some form of a healthy breakfast, a piece of fruit or a bowl of oatmeal, sometimes followed by a cup of coffee, but not every day.

Benefits of water, stretching, and meditation include, but are not limited to:

- Quenching the body's need for fluid, in the form of water.

- Allowing adrenal glands to naturally get going, versus a major kick in the rear.

- Preventing muscles and ligaments from shortening; that shortening leads to tightening and tension later in life.

- Creating a visualization of the day ahead through quiet, centering time.

- Developing improved self-confidence through inner reflection.

Now I'm ready to face the outside world, even though it's all from my home office. The above routine has some flexibility and, once established, takes only thirty to sixty minutes. Starting your day this way will set a positive tone and become a habit that will be missed if not done many times a week.

"Distraction Syndrome"

In my experience, if the first thing done to start the day is checking email or Facebook announcements, often the remainder of that day will be filled with the same. Plus, there's the lure of what I like to call Distraction Syndrome—DS. Once you get on the web, chances are you're going to be seduced. It's never easy to go on the internet for one simple thing without being pulled in other directions. Just don't do it!

Time Management

Time management is an essential part of completing necessary tasks without introducing more stress to your day. Placing strict time limits on particular tasks or extracurricular activities, such as web surfing, helps keep you on track and focused. I like to set up a simple to-do list with a time frame attached, such as whether a task will be completed in the morning or afternoon. Unless there is a need for more specific timing, such as getting kids to school or attending a meeting, clumping activities into morning, afternoon, or evening yields a sense of structure and accomplishment. It's a great feeling to mark items off my list as I complete my daily tasks.

This process only relieves stress as long as the to-do list isn't overly ambitious. For this method to be helpful, it also needs to be realistic. Placing too many items on this list and not getting them all done only adds to the stress level at the end of your day.

2

Computer Vision Syndrome

BLURRY VISION AT THE END OF THE DAY

Symptoms often occur after reading, long hours of computer work, or other close activities that involve tedious visual tasks.

Computer Vision Syndrome is a form of eye strain, which is a condition that causes nonspecific symptoms such as fatigue, pain in or around the eyes, blurred vision, bloodshot eyes, headaches, and occasionally double vision.

Our eyeballs are a complex arrangement of nerves and fluids. Eye movement and sight are controlled by eye muscles, eight per eye, that determine which direction you look. The shape of the eyeball has a lot to do with whether someone has 20/20 vision or is near- or farsighted, and the muscles that control eye movement also are responsible for how eyeballs are shaped. Eyeballs are housed in eye sockets, and muscles around the eye sockets are responsible for maintaining their shape. Imagine a softball in a glove, where the softball would be the eyeball and the glove would be the eye socket.

When you look at something at close range, like a computer screen two to three feet away, it causes eye muscles to contract, pulling the eyeball closer to the lens. When looking at something far away, twenty feet or more, the eye muscles relax, which allows the eyeball to move farther from the lens. If you were to clench your fist and hold that clench for an hour, or even for a few minutes, you might experience muscle spasms or soreness in your hand. Eye muscles can go through a very similar process. They get exhausted, which is why after hours of close visual work, you might experience headaches, blurred vision, bloodshot eyes, and many other symptoms.

Let's say you work at your computer between four and eight hours per day, which does not include an average of 2.6 hours of personal computer time. That means eye muscles are in a contracted state that whole time. As more time is spent looking at our computer monitors, tablets, e-readers, and smartphones (internet use has increased about 121% since 2009), the complaints associated with computer-related injuries, small-screen eye strain, and computer vision syndrome are increasing. Small-screen eye strain indicates that eyes have been looking at a small screen at close range for long periods of time and have become strained.

Continuing to subject our eyes to small screens leads to eye strain, eventually causing fatigue of the eye muscles, which then leads to symptoms—headaches, loss of focus, blurred vision, double vision, and neck and shoulder pain. This is particularly true for tablet, smartphone, and e-reader users. I'm not suggesting you stop using these devices; they have become part of our lives and are not likely to be disappearing anytime soon. What I am recommending is finding a balance and integrating some healthy habits that help maintain better eye health.

One recommendation is implementing the 20/20/20 rule.

1. Every 20 minutes.
2. Stop looking at the screen and look at an object at least 20 feet away.
3. Focus on that object for at least 20 seconds.

This not only rests your eyes from small-screen strain but also relaxes the muscles of the eye. A mere twenty seconds gives eye muscles a break from having been in a contracted state the whole time you were focused on your monitor.

Another situation we must contend with is being in air conditioning most of the day. Dry air and lack of adequate hydration, added to constant eye strain, can exacerbate another eye condition: xerophthalmia, or dry eyes. Air conditioning and closed windows also contribute to what is called Sick Building Syndrome, which is a list of symptoms caused by recirculation of non-filtered air.

Poor air quality, poor circulation, and the drying effects of cool, conditioned air lead to tear ducts drying out. Although this tends to be temporary while in the building or office, effects can be irritating. Tears help keep the eyes clean and flushed as well as moistened. One of the reasons we blink is to activate the tear

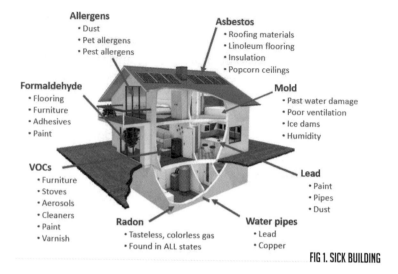

Allergens
- Dust
- Pet allergens
- Pest allergens

Asbestos
- Roofing materials
- Linoleum flooring
- Insulation
- Popcorn ceilings

Formaldehyde
- Flooring
- Furniture
- Adhesives
- Paint

Mold
- Past water damage
- Poor ventilation
- Ice dams
- Humidity

VOCs
- Furniture
- Stoves
- Aerosols
- Cleaners
- Paint
- Varnish

Lead
- Paint
- Pipes
- Dust

Radon
- Tasteless, colorless gas
- Found in ALL states

Water pipes
- Lead
- Copper

FIG 1. SICK BUILDING

ducts, which causes tears to flow to moisten the eyes. Blinking can aid in keeping our eyes hydrated. Eyes, like any other body tissue or system, rely on good nutrition and hydration as well as, yes, it is true, exercise.

Vitamin A and Your Eyes

When it comes to nutrition, eyes are dependent on a few significant vitamins and minerals. Without these vital ingredients, which include antioxidants, eye health can degenerate over time. One substance well known to support eye health is vitamin A. Not eating or taking an adequate dose on a regular basis leads to a deficiency.

A symptom of vitamin A deficiency that is easily reversible is slow light accommodation. When you walk from a room with ample light into a dark room, it should only take about ten seconds for your eyes to adjust. If it takes longer than thirty seconds, you could have a vitamin A deficiency. Consuming vitamin A most often resolves this issue.

Another vitamin A deficiency symptom is long-standing dry eyes and difficulty focusing your sight. This is not to say that vitamin A is the sole cause if there is a change in your vision, but it's worth exploring along with a visit to an optometrist.

Vitamin A has several important functions in the body, so it's great we actually have a benign warning signal when there's a deficiency. Take heed of the warning early, and you won't find yourself stranded on the side of the road at night, unable to adjust to changing light conditions.

Fortunately, many fruits and vegetables are good sources of beta carotene, which our bodies convert to vitamin A. The most familiar of these is carrots, but beta carotene, a precursor to vitamin A, is also present in sweet potatoes, pumpkin squash, mango, spinach, cantaloupe, and kale. While sitting at the computer and deciding what you're going to snack on, consider a sweet potato, kale chips, dried vegetable chips, or a bowl of cantaloupe, which will add nutrition to your diet without adding too many calories. There are many ways to make this bright variety of foods tasty and exciting, which prevents monotony and taste-bud boredom. More of this will be covered in a later chapter.

Position, Position, Position

In addition to exercises, hydration and nutrition, proper position and ergonomics can help avert eye strain. There are several key elements to consider.

The positioning of your monitor is extremely important because the screen is what you will be looking at for hours. Place the monitor at a height where you don't have to lean your head forward or tilt it downward. Ideally, position the monitor so that your nose aligns with the center of the screen. This way, you don't have to bend your neck and are able to maintain proper alignment of your head and spine, which relieves tension in the neck and shoulder muscles. While sitting at your desk using a desktop computer, choose a larger screen, ideally seventeen or nineteen inches (larger if available). This helps reduce eye strain and allows for more distance between you and the screen.

A good starting point is to have the monitor at least an arm's length away. Also crucial is screen resolution—a high pixel count per inch. This provides better picture quality, making for a clearer image. None of these features means having to spend a lot of money these days. I recommend trying to view the monitor in use before purchasing so you can see if it is a proper fit for you. For those who use tablets, e-readers, and smartphones a lot, remembering the 20/20/20 rule is your best defense against eye strain and posture problems. Regarding positioning of these devices, make sure that you shift your position frequently, whether lying on a couch or sitting in a lounge chair or whatever piece of furniture you've chosen.

Proper positioning is important because the screens on these gadgets emit a type of light that is not best suited for eye health with long-term use. If possible, position your monitor so you are facing open space in a room or office. This lets you look up and away regularly, thus giving your eyes the break they need from close viewing. Placing the monitor against a wall limits your ability to look up and away without getting up or turning your chair around. When your desk and monitor face outward, even if you are focused on the work at hand, peripheral vision still offers your eyes the ability to take in other images. This not only has benefits for the eyes but also contributes to relaxing your brain from such strenuous focus. Sticky notes can be used to remind you to take regular visual breaks. I place them on my monitor to remind me to look away every twenty minutes and to sit up straight—posture is also important! Looking at something in the distance should be done for twenty seconds, which is enough time to relax those contracted eye muscles. If you find this starts turning into ten to twenty minutes, you may want to consider a vacation!

Proper lighting can make a significant difference in how your eyes feel at the end of the day. Direct lighting that doesn't produce a glare on the screen and provides some flexibility—such as a swivel or adjustable desk lamp—is what I suggest. Ambient or track lighting is the most effective in providing the light necessary without glare.

Your desk chair, considering the amount of time you will sit at your desk, should be an investment worth your weight in gold. An adequate chair, otherwise known as your desk throne, will

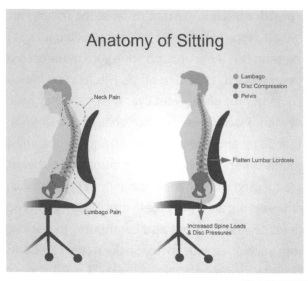

FIG 2. ANATOMY OF SITTING

supply multiple height adjustments, lumbar back support, and adjustable armrests. If you don't have the finances on hand now, a decent chair is worth saving for. Until then, you can use home-made attachments: a lumbar roll for low back support, cushions for seat positioning, padding for armrests, and so on.

Leg and foot health is just as important while sitting long hours. A foot stool, foot roller, or wooden foot massager could be used while sitting, thus accomplishing a foot massage while elevating the feet one to three inches off the floor. This stimulates foot and leg movement, which contributes to increased circulation in the lower legs and feet.

Crossing your legs for long hours puts strain on blood vessels in the lower legs and behind the knees. It also causes a twisting effect on the pelvis and a stretching effect on muscles and tendons of the outer thighs. Over time, this position can lead to lowered circulation in the legs and feet. Because lymphatic vessels (they're like blood vessels but carrying lymph fluid) are near the surface, crossing legs when sitting for long periods also hinders lymph flow, which is part of why feet and ankles swell. Those who use tablets and e-readers need to think about posture when sitting in a lounge chair or couch for several hours. If you can get lost in the internet or in a good book, allow yourself and your body the respect of moving around and changing position on a regular basis. Find a new position, or at least move around before settling back into your lounge chair or couch.

Computer Vision Syndrome is a list of symptoms associated with long hours of staring at a monitor (including tablets, smartphones, and e-readers): burning eyes, dry eyes, headache, etc. It can be avoided by performing eye muscle exercises. Don't panic; this does not mean going to a special eye gym. These exercises can be done just about anywhere, except while driving! It takes approximately one to two minutes to perform a set of these exercises, and I recommend doing these a couple of times a day—at the very least when you feel your eyes getting tired. Following this simple sequence will engage the full range of motion that eyes have, which allows them to move in all eight directions. Exercising each of the separate muscles responsible for these eight movements allows the eyes to relax.

- Picture a clock while keeping your head straight and still. Moving only your eyes, look up at twelve, down to six, right to three, and left to nine. Then look to two o'clock, down to eight o'clock, up to ten o'clock, then down to four o'clock. Hold each position for five to seven seconds, and breathe as you're in each position. Inhale, look in the designated direction, and then slowly release your breath while moving your eyes back to neutral. That's it.

- When the sequence is completed, cup your hands and place them over your eyes to block all light from entering, or as much as you can. This may sound funny, but while the eyes are in darkness, try to look out through your cupped hands. This relaxes the visual center of the brain while relieving the tension that can lead to low-grade headaches.

- These exercises can be done before, during, or after computer work. A good habit to incorporate is:
  - before starting your work
  - just before a lunch break
  - at the end of the day before (not while!) driving home.

Remember, it only takes sixty to ninety seconds, and your eyes will thank you.

Blue Light

Blue light wavelengths used to only come from the sun, which meant we were only exposed to them during daylight hours. Its shorter wavelengths have higher energy output and are stronger than red or green on a light scale. Beneficial during daylight hours, blue light has been shown to boost attention, reaction times, and mood. However, blue light is disruptive at night. The increased use of electronics with screens; i.e., smartphones, tablets, laptops, plus more energy-efficient lighting, is increasing our exposure to blue wavelengths, especially after sundown. We do know that this suppresses the secretion of melatonin, a hormone that influences circadian rhythms, in addition to having other ill effects on hunger, sleep patterns, and eye health.

A Harvard study showed a potential connection between blue light and diabetes, and possibly obesity. The researchers put ten people on a schedule that gradually shifted the timing of their circadian rhythms. Their blood sugar levels increased, throwing them into a prediabetic state, and levels of leptin, a hormone that leaves people feeling full after a meal, went down.

Blue light also has been connected to digital eye strain, contributing to fatigue, dry eyes, sore or irritated eyes, headaches, and difficulty focusing. The use of phones, with their smaller screens, has been shown to cause more strain.

Because of the patterns and practices of modern life, humans are not exposed to adequate levels of natural light during the day. They are, however, overexposed to artificial light at night. Current research shows that overexposure to blue light, mostly at night, can lead to different levels of damage in the eyes and skin.

Studies suggest continued exposure to increased amounts of blue light, over time, could lead to damage of the retina— the layer of light-sensitive cells at the back of the eye that pass impulses to the optic nerve.

The increased use of light-emitting diodes (LEDs) and the significantly increased use of smartphones, tablets, laptops, and desktop computers show that exposure of human skin cells to LEDs from electronic devices, even for periods of time as short as one hour, may cause damage to skin, eyes, and normal sleep patterns. The skin is a major target of oxidative stress, also known as free radical damage, and the link between aging and this free radical damage has been well studied.

Simple Solutions:

- For your eyes, investigate saline eye drops to combat dryness from air-conditioned environments and prolonged screen use. Placing a humidifier or essential oil diffuser near your desk can also add moisture to the air.

- Position your computer screen twenty-eight to forty inches from your face, and adjust its position so that your gaze is directed slightly downward. Remember the 20/20/20 rule—every twenty minutes, look at something twenty feet away for twenty seconds.

- Taking breaks and reducing the amount of screen time is optimal, but there are physical aids you can use to reduce the impact of screen time on your eyes. Computer glasses with yellow-tinted lenses can block blue light and increase contrast, helping to alleviate eye strain. Anti-reflective lenses can also reduce glare, block blue light, and increase contrast. If you want blue-light filters that aren't perched on your nose, there are screen filters available for smartphones, tablets, and computer screens.

Hydration

I cannot stress enough the importance of adequate fluids—primarily filtered water, hot or cold tea, and diluted fruit juice. If you look forward to the occasional bubbles of a soda, I recommend making your own. By combining six ounces of carbonated water with two ounces of quality fruit juice, you can make the equivalent of a healthy soda. The difference here is you have controlled the amount of sugar and did not include any preservatives. This recipe also may wind up saving you money compared with the cost of canned soda.

One of the biggest challenges I found with most of my patients was their ability to keep track of how much water they drank on any given day. I'll be honest; it's not easy to remember what I had for breakfast some mornings, much less how many cups of water I drank in a day.

Simple Solution: Use a premeasured container.

- Using a quart-size glass jar or insulated bottle ensures you're getting at least thirty-two ounces of water without having to think too much about it. Just fill it in the morning and know that you need to finish it before the end of the workday. (And thirty-two ounces of coffee or soda doesn't count. They have a diuretic effect, meaning they cause more water loss than what they contribute.)

- A single, average can of soda has seven to nine teaspoons of sugar, which contributes considerably to the amount of sugar consumed in a day. If you don't care for the taste of water, and some people don't, try filtered water or even adding some mild flavoring like lemon, lime, or a splash of juice. Besides keeping the body hydrated, water contributes to preventing the tear ducts from drying out. It also gives you a good reason to take more short breaks—trips to the restroom. These restroom breaks might seem too interrupting, but remember it's a good thing to move and get out of the chair regularly. I recommend doing it at least every hour, even if that means just standing up at your desk and stretching—rolling shoulders back, moving your neck and head around, and stretching your wrists are three common forms of exercises that are easy to integrate into a one- to two-minute break.

Nutrition Specifics

It would be great if we could meet all our nutritional needs with a healthy and balanced diet, but our modern-day lifestyle demands more than our modern-day food can supply. I believe our country's growing obesity rates, including that of our children, are in part due to poor quality, high-calorie, sugary or fatty foods. We also are sitting much more and are considerably less active than prior generations. This combination is proving detrimental to our health.

While sitting at my desk, I'm often looking for some easy food or snack to satisfy my desire for crunch and flavor. There are options that can accomplish these cravings without contributing a lot of extra calories. One example is slicing an apple and putting peanut butter or almond butter on several of the slices. This provides both the crunch factor and a satisfying snack that requires about two minutes to prepare. It's also easy to eat while continuing to work at the computer, with there being little mess to deal with.

Multitasking! This buzzword has earned its place in our schedules, much like breathing and sleeping. Thinking about many things at once demands higher octane fuel to run our "jet engines," our brains. This seems the perfect time to introduce quality supplements. Not all supplements are created equal—a fancy label or a steep price does not necessarily indicate quality ingredients. Attempting to save money by purchasing a supplement that has twenty-three ingredients does you no favors either. Quality ingredients mean quality supplements, and when we're talking about our eyes, quality matters. Quality supplements do usually cost more due to the cost of the ingredients, but it's worth it in the long run.

Simple Solution: Ah, the Smoothie

One approach when considering sources for concentrated nutrition is vegetable juicing and smoothies.

- Juicing and smoothies allow for taking in a greater number of vitamins and minerals without adding significant calories. I recommend using color variation when choosing fruits and vegetables. This ensures a good array of vitamins and minerals while preventing taste-bud boredom. There is nothing worse than getting bored with food that's good for you.

- When making smoothies, change the fruit or flavor enhancers used—the type of juice as the liquid portion (apple, blueberry, pomegranate), powdered protein mixes, or other such ingredients. A suggestion is to freeze fruit, or buy frozen, to use instead of ice to avoid diluting your smoothie.

- Vegetable juicing packs nutrition into something that's easy to drink while sitting at your desk. When juicing, it's a good idea to mix in watery vegetables—cucumber, celery, zucchini, and beets. Apples add a nice flavor, some sweetness or tang depending on the variety used. Another benefit to juicing is enough juice can be made to last one to two days, which simplifies preparation. Keep it longer than that, however, and the juice starts to break down and lose its flavor and nutritional benefits. There are many good recipes available for fruit smoothies and vegetable juicing. Let your taste buds be your guide.

Recap:

- Take regular breaks from staring at any screen; remember the 20/20/20 rule.

- Performing eye muscle exercises will strengthen and relax the eyes.

- Water, water, water.

- Health supplements—whether capsules, tablets, or food—will add nutrients needed for the increased demand on the eyes and brain.

3

Headaches, Neck Tension

A BOWLING BALL ON YOUR SHOULDERS

This expression is used to classify headaches, stiff muscles, and tightness of the neck, typically resulting from a person using a computer over an extended period of time, or prolonged use in an inefficient manner.

Have you ever had a tension headache—a pain in the neck (not referring to your job) where it felt like the weight of the world was on your shoulders? Neck and shoulder pain is common today. It has some distinguishing characteristics that are often triggered by common causes. Gaining insight into what provokes these symptoms will better equip you to make adjustments that can correct the aggravating causes. The human head weighs ten to twelve pounds (or 4.5–5.2 kilograms), approximately eight percent of our body weight. That's about the weight of a novice's bowling ball.

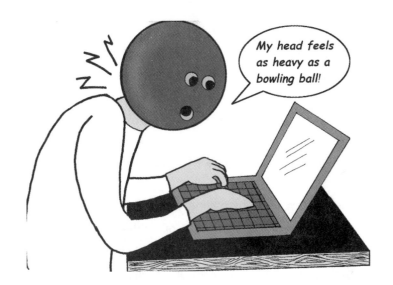

FIG 3. BOWLING BALL

When you consider all the components that make up the human head: bones, fluids, soft tissue, and so on, it's easy to see how the head weighs what it does. If it wasn't for the superb engineering of the body—we must thank the designer—the weight of our head would constantly cause us balance problems. We would look inebriated, a state that actually does throw our balance off.

How is this prevented? By an elaborate system of muscles and tendons in the neck and upper back that holds our head precisely in place, attached to our shoulders, maintaining constant balance. For the head to be tilted in one direction, some muscles contract, or pull and shorten, while other muscles lengthen while staying taut. Opposing muscles doing their job allow your head to tilt and turn in a controlled manner, preventing it from just flopping over.

If you've ever played tug of war, you will have a good idea how muscles in the body work. Each team involved in the game is trying to pull the other team over the center. Imagine if there were only one team pulling on the rope without resistance from an opposing team. The game would be over rather quickly—and not much fun. With certain muscles pulling while other muscles offer resistance, there is a controlled movement.

You should now see why having your head tilted forward at a computer screen for many hours, or holding a phone against your ear, leads to tension in the neck and shoulders. The muscles that are holding your head up are like the group of people trying not to let their group be pulled across the dead zone. Maintaining this constant position is referred to as static contraction. After one or more hours with their head in the same position, it's no wonder people complain of a pain in the neck.

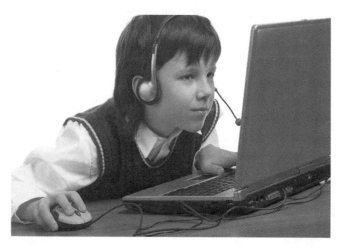

FIG 4. HEAD POSITION

Static contraction is not solely reserved for the computer operator. Similar principles apply to tablet, smartphone, and e-reader users. Circulation is improved by movement, and anytime someone spends long hours in a fixed posture, they experience a decrease in healthy circulation. Whenever I'm in a bad mood, I blast some music and dance around for a while. Just the act of moving my body and circulating more blood lifts my mood and shifts my attitude. To give you an idea of how important movement is, patients confined to bed rest for long periods of recovery are instructed to move as much and as often as possible to ameliorate their risk of developing bedsores.

I am not saying you're going to develop chair sores from sitting for many hours, but the principles are the same. Active muscles generate heat, which must be eliminated by the body's cooling system—perspiring and breathing—or overheating will occur. Body temperature is maintained, in large part, by the activity of muscle contraction. Static muscle contraction also has the tendency to cause muscle spasms or tension, which can lead to tension headaches or, for some people, migraines.

One particular cause of neck and shoulder pain is the buildup of acid in active muscles. Acidosis is a waste product of muscle contraction—especially when there is strain; as in long hours at an office desk. As this acid level rises in your muscles and is not eliminated by movement, it adds to discomfort.

Another function of water is to aid in the removal of the acid, helping to eliminate it from neck and shoulder muscles. Water flushes this waste product into the bloodstream. Once waste is in circulation, there are mechanisms that help to neutralize the acid, making it more alkaline. As an analogy, imagine throwing a leaf into a flowing stream, where the stream is like a blood vessel, the water like our blood, and the leaf would be the acid. If waste is flowing in circulation, our body can deal more easily with it. Pressure points or trigger points are, because of this waste buildup, causing muscles to tense, thus creating pain.

Our bodies know how to deal with elevated acid levels, to a point. But when this acid level is elevated for long periods of time, it interferes with other normal functions. Examples of this interference would be poor digestion and excess gas, occasional abnormal heart rate, blood sugar imbalances, and many more. Our body's pH, or acid/alkaline level, is even more tightly controlled than our body temperature. Stress is a huge contributor to altering blood pH or elevating blood acid levels. Even after thirty-one years in health and wellness, I am still awed by the fine balance required by the human body to maintain health. While we are resilient in many ways, the number of people each year who visit doctors' offices and hospitals for conditions that are often preventable indicates that even our resilience has its limits.

Water and Stretching

Water

I cannot stress enough the importance of drinking clean, preferably filtered water throughout the day. Water plays so many roles in our body, from diluting certain chemicals, aiding waste elimination, detoxifying, and reducing heat from normal muscle activity to lubricating your joints and many more. Just as oil in our car is important for lubricating moving parts, or fluid in a radiator for keeping the motor cool, water is that important to our bodies. There has been much debate around how much water a person should drink in a day, but not all water has to come from drinking. Fresh fruits and vegetables can count for a portion of water intake.

Several markers help in determining a person's water needs. Thirst is one, but it shouldn't be totally relied on; some people actually lose their ability to notice thirst. I worked with an office manager who would go all day without drinking water and vow she wasn't even thirsty at the end of her shift. (Personally, I think she was part camel without the hump.) A simple general test for determining a body's hydration status is called tenting. Place your palm on a flat surface. Relax the hand and, with your other hand, gently pinch some skin on the back of your flattened hand. Release the pinched skin and watch how it returns to its normal position. If you are well hydrated, your skin should return to normal within approximately one second. If it takes longer, there's a good chance you're not drinking enough water. This is just a general test, but it is quite useful.

Stretching

Stretching also plays a vital role in relaxing wrists, hands, and neck and shoulder muscles. In this case, we're not talking about a full yoga routine, just simple stretches that can be done at your desk. Over time with poor posture, muscles, tendons, and ligaments change their shape. Having your shoulders rolled forward for many hours of computer work, or your head bent sideways as with holding a phone, will eventually cause particular muscles and tendons to shorten. The change in muscle length causes muscle groups to be in a more contracted state (shortened) or a stretched-out state (lengthened). Either way, this doesn't affect tendons or muscles in the short term. But long term—say hours a day for weeks, months, or years—it can have a considerable effect on the anatomy.

Preventing muscle shortening is easier and less painful than treating it. Incorporating a stretching routine should not cause more pain than it relieves when regularly done. I like the rule of "three by seven": stretching in a particular direction three times, holding each stretch for seven seconds. This allows the muscles to relax and stay stretched out. Longer durations are better, but they may not be practical at work—unless your boss joins you, or you are the boss!

Simple Solutions: Stretching exercises!

With simple performance of these stretches on a consistent basis, many complaints of headaches, neck and shoulder tension, and upper back problems could be avoided or greatly reduced. This yields a healthier experience while at the computer or tablet, and a happier body to boot. This simple stretching routine can extend the relationship you have with your computer without sacrificing your health.

- **Head tilt:** Keeping your shoulders parallel with your hips, take a deep breath. As you exhale, tilt your head backward so your nose points toward the ceiling. Inhale and return to neutral. Repeat this two more times. Next, tilt your head forward, maintaining neutral shoulder position. Repeat three times.

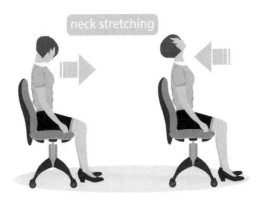

FIG 5. HEAD TILT

- **Neck stretch:** Inhale while sitting up straight, shoulders back and relaxed, exhale, and tip your head toward one shoulder and hold for seven seconds. Take a breath and return to a neutral position. Repeat this two more times. Then stretch in the opposite direction, for a total of three times with a seven-second hold, breathing each time.

- **Neck rotation:** Keep shoulders back and relaxed. Take a deep breath and, as you exhale, rotate your head as if looking over your left shoulder. There's no need to stress this stretch too much, as each time you perform this stretch you should notice greater rotation with an easing of tension. Perform this stretch three times and then repeat this to the right shoulder.

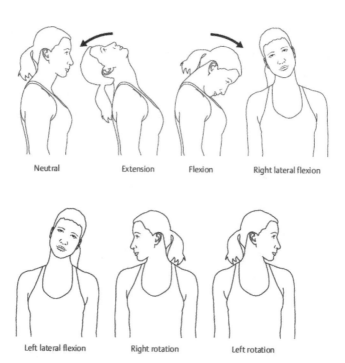

Neutral   Extension   Flexion   Right lateral flexion

Left lateral flexion   Right rotation   Left rotation

FIG 6. NECK STRETCH

- **Neck flexion:** Starting from a neutral position, take a deep breath, exhale, and tilt your head sideways as if you were trying to touch your shoulder with your ear. It's important here to keep your shoulders straight while bending your head. Remember that this is not an Olympic event. Just relax into this stretch. Hold this stretch for seven seconds and repeat two more times, then switch to the other side. This whole routine should take about two minutes, just enough time to relax the neck and shoulders without interfering with your work.

Relaxing tension in the neck and shoulders can help prevent afternoon tension headaches, improve your breathing, and increase work efficiency, so the boss shouldn't object

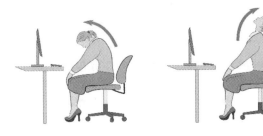

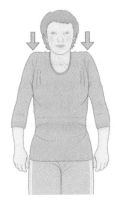

FIG 7. NECK FLEXION

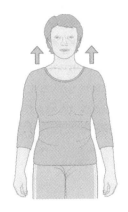

FIG 8. SHOULDER STRETCH

to this short break. When you have finished stretching, it's a good idea to drink a full glass of water. I suggest doing this a couple of times per day, especially if you are at a desk for five to eight hours. This could also be done on a lunch break.

- **Shoulder stretch and roll:** Begin by sitting up with your shoulders parallel to hips. Take a deep breath, exhale, and firmly but gently raise your shoulders as if trying to touch your ears without letting the shoulders roll forward. Hold this position for several seconds. Then inhale while relaxing them down. There is a tendency to let the head shrink into your shoulders. Remember, you're not trying to see how close you can get your shoulders to your ears; you are just stretching out certain shoulder muscles. I like to place my hands on my thighs while doing this stretch as it offers some support as well as guides me through proper movement.

- **Backward shoulder roll:** Place your hands on your thighs, inhale, and raise the shoulders up, holding for two to three seconds. Exhale while rolling shoulders backward, extending the chest forward. Relax back to neutral and repeat two to three more times.

- **Forward shoulder roll:** This is performed the same way, except start by raising the shoulders upward, followed by rolling them forward and then back to starting position. Always remember to breathe. Voila—you're all done!

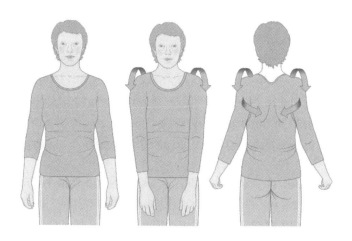

FIG 9. SHOULDER ROLL

- **Massage and bodywork:** What used to be considered a luxury is proving to be extremely beneficial for body, mind, and brain function. Even a fifteen-minute chair massage once or twice a month, which can be done in the office, has far-reaching benefits. A chair massage is done fully clothed and can be done in a public place. This type of bodywork can improve well-being and ease tension among employees. This also may come with increased productivity, a positive effect on attitude, and as a bonus for employers, a morale boost for employees. If you are inclined to recommend this to the boss, the cost-benefit ratio is likely to be good—not to mention it's rare for employees to miss work on Massage Day.

4

HANDS-DOWN PAINFUL

Carpal Tunnel Syndrome (CTS): A disorder caused by compression at the wrist of the median nerve supplying the hand, causing numbness and tingling.

There is a nerve that passes from the neck in the shoulder area down the arm and through a type of tunnel in your wrist. (Actually, there are several nerves that follow this path.) At the wrist, these nerves are bundled together, and they then pass through the "carpal tunnel," which received its name because the bones in our wrists are called carpal bones. Surrounding this nerve bundle is a protective sheath—very much like the material that covers wires in any electrical cord you have in your home. The sheath's main function is keeping the nerves together and protected from friction in the wrist. With long hours of use in a poorly positioned hand, due to the bad design of most keyboards and the computer mouse, stress is placed on these nerves. Constant stress on this nerve bundle leads to irritation, which, if continued, leads to inflammation.

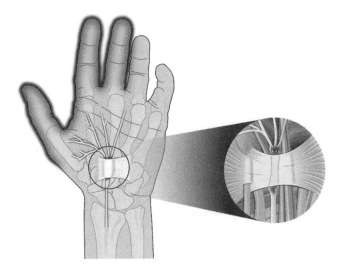

FIG 10. CTS

When our body detects inflammation, our immune system kicks into action. As a first line of defense, various chemicals are produced that are directed to the area of inflammation, leading to swelling. Swelling, an accumulation of fluids that acts as a protective mechanism, creates a cushion around the area of inflammation in an attempt to limit further damage or injury. This is like an airbag inflating in a car to protect drivers and passengers in a crash.

If what caused the initial irritation and swelling continues, like typing or handling a poorly designed mouse for hours at a time, the swelling increases. This increased pressure on the nerve bundle leads to tingling, pain, and eventually numbness. By not taking regular breaks and stretching muscles, tendons, and ligaments in the forearms and wrists, it becomes almost impossible for healing to occur. If the activity continues, nerve damage will occur, which often leads to a more serious need for intervention. One such treatment would be surgery to alleviate the pressure caused by the swelling. Nerves are slow to recover and require long periods of rehab and rest.

This is where prevention could save a lot of suffering and time lost from work or life activities. In many cases, just stopping the activity that caused the initial aggravation for a period of time (days to weeks) can lead to healing and recovery. In the case of a carpenter swinging a hammer for many hours or a computer operator typing for long hours, the body cannot get enough reprieve for healing to happen without adequate rest. Realistically, this often is not an option when these activities are part of your job. There are many cases of carpal tunnel reported each year that cause lost work time and income.

If your boss makes accommodations for your recovery, there is the issue of what to do to accomplish it. Physical therapy, occupational therapy, acupuncture, massage, and, mostly, the rest required to recuperate would all be in your plan of recovery. The problem is that when you return to work at the same task that caused the trouble in the first place, you are right back where you started. Luckily, there are activities that can be incorporated into your workplace that don't require much expense or time off.

Repetitive strain injuries (RSIs) are "injuries of the musculoskeletal and nervous systems that may be caused by repetitive tasks, forceful exertions, vibrations, mechanical compression (pressing against hard surfaces), or sustained or awkward positions."[1].

RSI problems are also known as cumulative trauma disorders, repetitive stress injuries, repetitive motion injuries or disorders, musculoskeletal disorders, and (occupational) overuse syndromes. Preventing carpal tunnel syndrome is a matter of a few simple techniques regularly applied and is often cheaper than rehab or lost time from work. As a result of many jobs or activities that require repetitive motion, including certain hobbies, a whole area of specially designed furniture, tools, and gadgets have been invented to ease pressures placed on our bodies. The Occupational Safety and Health Administration (OSHA) defines ergonomics as "...the science of fitting workplace conditions and job demands to the capabilities of the working population." This "fit" includes arranging the environment in which you work to prevent injury and increase productivity.

In terms of a computer workstation, ergonomics refers to the physical position at which you sit at your computer, the ventilation in the area, and the effectiveness and safety of direct and ambient lighting. Psychology, biomechanics, kinesiology, and other factors are also considered when enhancing our efficiency and relieving stress on our bodies. An example of this is the keyboard. By using a traditional keyboard that has all the keys in straight lines, our hands and wrists are forced into an unnatural position. For a short time, most people wouldn't feel the effects, but after long hours of repetitive work, day after day, week after week, this position begins to take its toll.

A straight-line keyboard design forces us to turn our hands slightly outward, meaning bent in a direction toward the pinky finger. Holding this position causes irritation in the wrists, specifically the nerves that travel through the carpal tunnel. Conversely, ergonomic keyboards are designed to place our wrists in a more natural position. Natural human position and body posture is referred to as our anatomical position. Try standing up straight, allowing your arms to hang by your sides with palms facing forward, thumb gently extended. Now observe how your wrists naturally fall. This is your anatomical position.

Maintaining anatomical position, bring your hands up and place them on your present keyboard. If done correctly, you should find the need to turn your wrists outward to accommodate traditional keyboard designs. An ergonomic keyboard, however, mimics how our wrists would fall naturally, thereby relieving strain on the carpal tunnel in the wrist. Better ergonomic keyboards also provide an elevated cushion for where your hands would be resting. A similar approach in design has been applied to a variety of tools: the computer mouse, monitors, certain equipment used in different industries, carpentry tools. Even kitchen utensils have incorporated ergonomic design technology.

Another example of where ergonomics would be applied is a desk chair. When considering the natural contours of your spine, the distance between the back of your thigh and your feet on the floor, and the armrests, you can see how most chairs place our body in a poor posture. This is especially significant if we sit for many hours at a time. An ergonomic chair offers areas of support in the lower back or lumbar region, adjustable armrests for better shoulder positioning, and adjustable seat height so our feet can reach the floor regardless of our height and leg length. Also, a chair's ventilation is important. After sitting for several hours against a leather or faux leather chair, heat can build up against your lower back. This can lead to lower back muscle fatigue.

Ergonomic design has not received the attention it deserves. Many tools are designed specifically to make our bodies and lives more attuned to the environment we work in—where we spend more time doing repetitive tasks. Implementing ergonomic design would mean less work time lost to certain avoidable injuries, which would mean less salary loss—not to mention less pain and suffering. It also would improve efficiency—getting more done in a shorter time. To illustrate, try using a dull pair of scissors to cut a large stack of paper. Then replace the dull scissors with a sharper pair and see how much

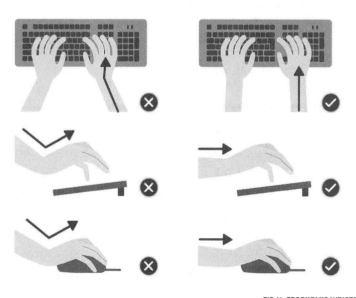

FIG 11. ERGONOMIC WRISTS

more quickly and easily the job gets done. Better tools at your job workstation or home office can improve performance.

Simple Solutions: Rest and Stretch

Remember, breathing is important while performing each of the following stretches.

- **Take regular breaks**: One way to relieve wrist stress is to take regular breaks. During these short breaks, incorporate wrist stretching to reduce your risk for carpal tunnel syndrome. Regular breaks refer to a two- to three-minute respite every twenty to thirty minutes.

- **Wrist exercises:** Interlace your fingers, take a deep breath, and, as you exhale, extend your arms straight out in front of you so your palms are facing out. Hold this position for several seconds and repeat two more times. This is good for the shoulders as well.

- **Wrist flexion:** Lift one elbow out to one side and bend your forearm so your hand comes closer to your face. Take a deep breath; while exhaling bend your hand so the fingers are pointing toward the floor. Apply mild pressure with your other hand to the bent wrist. Hold this position for a count of five, then release. Repeat two more times.

- **Wrist extension:** Start by placing hands together in front of your chest with your fingers pointing up toward the ceiling. With your right hand, grab your left fingers and bend them

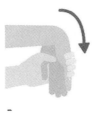

FIG 12. WRIST FLEXION

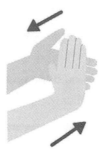

FIG 13. WRIST EXTENSION

back toward your elbow. Do not feel as though you have to push hard; a gentle pressure will do. Breathe and hold this for five seconds, then release. Switch and do the other hand the same way. Alternate between wrist flexion and extension as needed to relieve tension in your wrists and increase blood flow and circulation.

- **Fist forming and finger spreading:** Begin by making a fist. Take a breath, squeeze, and hold for two to three seconds. Exhale while you open your fist. Spread your fingers as wide as possible, hold position for two to three seconds. Repeat this motion several times. This exercise will increase

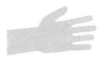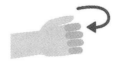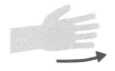

circulation in your hands and fingers while stretching and relaxing muscles and tendons.

- **Piano fingers:** With fingers extended, pretend to play the piano. Go crazy here if you want, especially if no one is watching! This could be done on a flat surface such as your desk, or in the air similar to air drumming or air guitar—but with more sophistication.

5

Circulation Complications

WHY DO MY LEGS, ANKLES, AND FEET SWELL?

Deep Vein Thrombosis (DVT): a blood clot in a deep vein, usually forming in legs, calves, or in the pelvic region.

Under normal conditions, our bodies form and dissolve blood clots quite often, after any kind of physical injury. The size of a clot mostly depends on the size of the injured area, and in some cases, we don't even know that a clot has formed. Anytime you bang your arm, shin, or other body part and get that typical black and blue mark, you have formed a type of clot. After repair of the damaged tissue, the immune system dissolves the clot, much like a clog in a kitchen sink gets dissolved with drain cleaner.

Most blood clots that form spontaneously occur in lower legs as a result of:

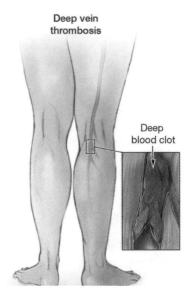

Deep vein
thrombosis

Deep
blood clot

FIG 15. DVT

1. Poor circulation.

2. Hyper-coagulability, or the increased tendency to form a clot.

3. Damage to a blood vessel wall.

There are many reasons for DVT or spontaneous clot formation—all of which can contribute to an increased health risk. Causes include, but are not limited to, pregnancy, trauma, hormone replacement therapy (HRT), obesity, older age and poor circulation, and immobilization. Long air travel (six to ten hours) and sitting for long periods without taking regular breaks are among the greatest risks.

Long airline flights increase clot risk because of the cramped quarters and lack of adequate leg movement, especially with a flight lasting six or more hours. Sitting still for so long creates a significant reduction of circulation in the feet, ankles, and legs. If there are any existing circulation problems, this can increase the chance of forming a clot. In people who do not have circulation problems, this is not usually an issue, as any clots that do form will spontaneously dissolve as readily as they were produced.

There are several warning signs to look for when discerning whether you are someone prone to forming spontaneous blood clots. Seeking medical attention is recommended if any of the following appear without cause, meaning there was no injury or accident that you can remember, if they appear suddenly, or if they last more than a couple of days.

1. Pain and tenderness in the lower leg without other known cause.

2. Swelling with pitting edema, meaning you press the swollen area and the indentation remains for five or more seconds.

3. Increased warmth in a particular area of the leg compared with the opposite leg or other body part.

4. Redness or discoloration without known cause or injury.

Comparing one leg with the other is good practice and serves as a point of reference. There are times when one leg could be affected and not necessarily the other. Performing a pitting edema self-test is a good way to assess how serious any swelling is.

Using a finger, push into the center of an area with swelling, remove your finger, and see how long it takes the indentation to return to normal. The longer the impression lasts, or the deeper the indentation is, the more important it is to seek further medical attention. Pitting edema could indicate a more serious condition and should not be ignored.

If the fingerprint resolves within a minute or so, this tends to indicate poor circulation. One of the causes is most likely prolonged sitting, which can be self-treated or prevented. On the other hand, if an area is discolored and has swelling, I recommend you see a medical health professional. Of greater concern are people in higher-risk categories: anyone with cardiovascular problems, lowered circulation, heart conditions, or pregnancy.

A clot in a deep vein of the leg can break off and travel to a smaller vessel in the lungs, heart, or brain. The traveling clot then becomes what is called an embolism, which can be life-threatening. Although it's not common for a clot to form in the lower leg of a healthy individual, it is always better to err on the side of safety and prevention. Since more and more people have sedentary work conditions—spending hours sitting at a computer desk—such clots could become more commonplace.

Prevention is Key

It costs much less to prevent an injury or health-related distress, when possible, than it does to treat it. Prevention also means less time lost at work, and lost time can mean loss of income—which adds to stress. By getting into good work habits and self-care, most foot, ankle, and leg swelling can be avoided.

1. 20/20/20 rule: While you're looking at something twenty feet away every twenty minutes to rest your eyes, do twenty seconds of leg and calf exercises.

2. Take a water or bathroom break every hour, preferably walking. This helps stimulate increased circulation in the lower legs.

3. Use a foot roller.

4. Wear graduated compression stockings.

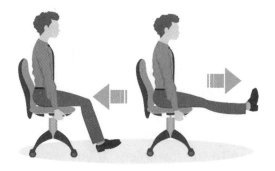

FIG 16. LEG AND CALF

Simple Solutions:

- **Leg and calf exercises:** While seated, extend both legs straight out and simultaneously point your toes forward, then flex your ankles. Rotate the feet in a circular motion, repeating several times. You can do one leg at a time if that is easier. If no one is watching, or you don't get embarrassed that easily, flap your legs as if swimming—just a few seconds will do. These exercises increase blood flow in your legs and cause you to change your posture during the exercise.

- **Water breaks:** Use these in much the same way a cigarette break was used in the past, but this being a healthier break. Simply walking to a water fountain (or the kitchen/refrigerator) will further two goals: drinking more water and increasing circulation, especially if the water source is a short walk from your desk.

- **Foot rollers:** These come in a variety of types and styles, meaning anything from inexpensive wooden rollers to electronic vibrating massagers. For this purpose, a simple wooden roller or platform roller is all that is needed. By pushing your foot across the floor on top of the roller, you accomplish several goals: 1) a foot massage that stimulates reflex points on the bottoms of your feet, and 2) movement that provides increased circulation to the lower legs. If you work in an office with others, it gives you an excuse to take your shoes off at work—as long as this doesn't anger your boss or co-workers.

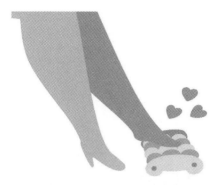

FIG 17. FOOT ROLLER

- **Graduated compression stockings:** These are specifically designed to lower the incidence of clots forming in the lower legs. By gradually decreasing the amount of pressure starting from the foot and ankle and extending up to the knee, they help increase blood flow back to the heart.

  Getting fitted with stockings that offer the correct amount of pressure is important. Improper fitting can cause additional circulation problems, which is what we are trying to avoid. Compression stockings aid in better blood flow, increased lymph flow, and maintaining warmth in the lower legs. These features are also beneficial for people who stand for long periods.

DVT, or deep vein thrombosis, is a condition that is preventable even for people whose job requires them to sit in front of a computer for long hours. Taking simple steps can protect and lower the risk of a blood clot forming in the most likely places—the lower legs and calves.

6

Mental Fatigue

BRAIN BURNOUT!

Mental fatigue is the result of brain overactivity; this is a condition where the brain cells become exhausted—much like our bodies do when we've been physically overactive.

Brain fog, clouded thinking, daydreaming, excessive yawning, and staring blankly into space are all signs of mental fatigue. Does this describe how you feel some days at your desk in front of your computer?

If you've ever physically worked out to a level of fatigue or been physically active for hours—such as chasing your children around or doing yard work—then you have experienced muscle exhaustion. Our brain cells are like muscles that have exhaustion levels, and this level is different for everyone. Each cell in the brain requires nutrition and adequate fluids to maintain optimal functioning. Think of your brain cells as little individual engines, where each one needs to be constantly fueled to keep running.

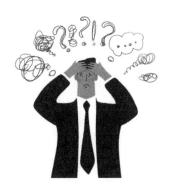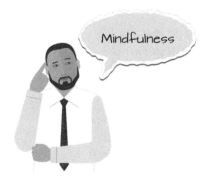

FIG 18. MENTAL OVERLOAD

One key difference between muscles and brain cells is that when most muscles get exhausted, they can just stop working for a short while until they recuperate. Our brains do not have this luxury. If any part of your brain just stopped working for a while, there would be serious consequences. Imagine if the part of your brain that controls breathing or heart rate decided it needed a ten-minute break, or the area of your brain that's responsible for seeing punched the time clock. Obviously, these are not options available to the brain.

In these times of multitasking, there is an above-average like-lihood that our brains will get overwhelmed. Our brains perform hundreds of thousands of functions on a daily basis, as all the information we process in our bodies has to be interpreted by the brain. This demand for continuous activity increases the need for periodic respites.

It was once thought that technology—computers, fax machines, internet, smartphones, and tablets—would simplify our lives. But instead of letting these machines just do some of our work, which they do, we've also let them increase the amount of work we do in a day. It's now easy to perform tasks while lying on the beach or sitting in a park. While we used to go to these places to relax, now we take our work with us and let laptops and smartphones consume a large part of this "relaxation" time with emails, texts, or even faxes.

With smartphones, we can now multitask without interrupting a phone call. Putting a call on speaker, we can also check email, send a text, and program a meeting on our calendar. Although our brain and nervous system can handle this activity, it is daunting. I have seen more adrenal fatigue, sleep problems, and digestion irregularities in the past five years than I did through the first ten years of my practice. I passionately believe there is a direct correlation between those conditions and advancing technology, and it's only getting worse.

Let's draw a picture to make this real: Here you are at your job, working on the computer. During this time, you are answering the phone and taking messages, scheduling appointments for upcoming meetings, and writing a to-do list of all the things you're going to accomplish that day and maybe the next day. In this mix, you are juggling family events and schedules and deciding what's going to be for dinner, which you will pick up on the way home after working out at the gym, hopefully. Somewhere in there is the chore of running several errands and squeezing in lunch, maybe. So far, this seems manageable but full. A flat tire or your car not starting, however, can throw a wrench into this well-planned list. Stress builds, and stress hormones get pumped into your body at alarming rates—which just adds more stress.

And this was a good day! If that scenario doesn't sound exhausting, then let's focus on the stress factor.

The Brain and Stress

Stress, a six-letter word that is somewhat misunderstood, is responsible for a multitude of health concerns. Mental stress stems from over-scheduling our daily lives on a regular basis. When we perceive how "stressed" we are, we often don't understand the cascade of stress hormones that are produced and secreted in our bodies. These hormones—cortisol, adrenaline, growth hormone, and others—cause certain reactions in the body, such as increased heart rate, poor digestion, decreased fat metabolism, increased body temperature, and many others.

The "fight or flight" response to stress is an innate reaction designed to help us handle stressful situations. If you saw your child about to do something that had harmful consequences, you would go into protective mode and respond within milliseconds, without even thinking about it. A type of "automatic pilot" takes over, and later you might wonder how you actually did what you did. Fight is your reaction to combat danger as quickly as possible, which is usually followed by a period of calm. Flight would be running from a burning building to save your life.

Our bodies were not designed to be in fight or flight mode for hours at a time. The response was designed to get us out of dangerous situations, quite possibly saving our lives, and then allow us to relax. During the fight or flight period, numerous hormones course through our body, and our brain is responsible for controlling all the goings-on. One big challenge with multitasking is that the brain does not differentiate well between danger and overstimulation/stress—both lead to the same hormones getting produced and secreted.

A patient came to see me with complaints of loss of focus, trouble concentrating, forgetting what she was doing—often walking into a room and forgetting why she went there. After taking her health history, I learned she was juggling two jobs amounting to twenty-five to thirty hours per week, a hospital rotation for nursing school that accounted for twenty to twenty-five hours per week, taking three academic classes, and doing her homework.

As we calculated the number of hours per week she was engaged in actual brain activity, she looked at me and said, "No wonder I'm so tired and can't focus." The effects of her schedule were so obvious to her boss one day that he sent her home out of concern for her well-being.

When we are so "maxed out," brain-wise, it becomes easy to make mistakes at work—or even more costly mistakes, such as not being able to focus while driving or performing some other type of potentially hazardous activity. I stopped counting how many of my patients had bruised or broken toes or shin wounds from walking into table legs, had cuts or burns from kitchen accidents, or had other injuries associated with loss of focus due to mental exhaustion.

Other symptoms of mental fatigue can include unexplained dizziness, lethargy—meaning you just don't feel like doing anything—lackluster attitude toward something you ordinarily enjoy, impaired long- and short-term recall (not to be confused with memory loss), and difficulty making decisions that usually didn't confound you in the past.

Short-term memory loss has become a serious issue among my patients and clients. I often hear complaints such as "I used to be able to do xyz with no problem, now I have trouble finding my keys." Or, "I find myself walking into a room and forgetting what I went in for." Have you ever found yourself driving someplace you have driven to a thousand times and forgetting how to get there, or calling a friend only to forget their name as soon as they answer the phone?

Chances are you have stress in your life—good stress and bad stress. Good stress gets us out of bed in the morning and helps us make certain decisions. I prefer to call it motivation, as in being motivated to get out of bed in the morning, or being motivated to start the day with breakfast. If, in fact, you knew that you would be managing more during your day by taking regular small breaks throughout the day, wouldn't you be motivated to include these breaks?

Bad stress, however, prompts your body to produce a hormone that handles it. That hormone, cortisol, causes your body to hold on to fat more readily, and it turns out that the type of fat that is retained appears to be more dangerous than regular body fat. It stores certain types of chemicals, including stress hormones.

More side effects of excessive cortisol are lowered mental capacity for thinking, poor sleep, and poor sleep patterns, all of which hinder clear thinking and mental performance. Cortisol also suppresses immune function and slows normal wound healing. That bad stress has a lot of side effects.

The Brain and Vitamin D

Another factor that may be contributing to people's mental exhaustion is a lack of vitamin D. Many people are spending most of their daytime hours indoors, which is contributing to deficiencies in the "sunshine vitamin," or vitamin D. Lately this deficiency is getting the attention it deserves. Vitamin D has behaviors that resemble hormone activity, and by looking at its functions in our body, we find that it acts in several systems.

Vitamin D is crucial for bone health. Significant vitamin D deficiency is directly linked to a condition in children known as rickets. Their bones don't harden properly, and one effect is that their legs are bowed. Vitamin D deficiency in adults leads to what is known as "soft bones," or osteomalacia. With adults, the soft bone condition increases the risk of broken bones and poor healing.

If vitamin D deficiency continues, it often contributes to the condition known as osteoporosis, in which the body's ability to regenerate new bone decreases. Our bodies make new bone throughout our lives; it is only when we don't do the things necessary to help this process along that bones weaken and break relatively easily later in life. A few actions undertaken on a regular basis can prevent much of this.

So, how does this connect with mental exhaustion? Vitamin D has effects on other areas of our health. Next time you have been sitting indoors for six hours and are feeling tired, take a break and go outside for ten minutes to sit in the sunshine. Natural sunlight shining on your eyes and your skin can markedly change your energy and mood. Simply exposing as much skin surface area, meaning arms, face, and possibly legs, to direct sunshine initiates some effects vitamin D has on other body systems. This is why some nutritionists liken vitamin D to a hormone.

My suggestion is to take short breaks outside daily, or every other day, and monitor how you feel at the end of a week. I have even prescribed a daily dose of sunshine to patients dealing with thyroid issues. One of the functions of our thyroid is to regulate an overall sense of well-being, and sunlight can improve the absorption of vitamin D—which adds to an overall feeling of wellness. Getting a daily dose of vitamin D from the sun, as opposed to a supplement, has made a significant difference in some of my patients' well-being. This "prescription" places sunshine into the therapeutic realm, with the only side effect being a slight tan.

The Brain and Time Breaks

Maintaining your focus hour after hour, especially while multi-tasking, becomes more and more challenging. During one of my classes at medical school, Dr. Fruehauf, the instructor, would require us to stop what we were doing every twenty to thirty minutes and take a one- to two-minute break. Often, he would just have us stand, stretch out our arms, and take a couple of deep breaths, then sit back down and get started where we'd left off. His contention was that the brain can only absorb so much intense information for a certain period of time. After that time limit had been reached, he told us, retention rates drop significantly. And he was right. Because Dr. Fruehauf allowed us a couple of minutes to absorb what we had just learned before going on, I found I had to study less for his class than I did for most of my other classes.

I equate this to taking a bite of food. Before eating the next bite, it's a good idea to chew and swallow the last bite well, thus allowing some digestion to take place between bites. By slowing down and taking short breaks between forkfuls of food, as with "forkfuls" of information, it often takes less food to reach a state of satisfaction and fullness.

There are a few ways, in addition to scheduling those short breaks throughout the day, you can adapt your office or home office environment to help battle bad stress.

First, organize. Have you ever been so busy that you had not gotten around to cleaning your kitchen, bathroom, or bedroom for too long? Then that day came when you whipped into action and became a cleaning machine. Remember how good it felt when you walked back into that room and saw everything in its place? At work, is your desk piled with papers, scribbled note-pads, files, and sticky notes? Take fifteen minutes and organize the chaos, and it will streamline your thought process and your work tasks for the day—or longer!

Second, surround yourself with things you love. When I was in school, I did some professional interior house painting with a friend to earn extra money. We began to incorporate faux finishing into our repertoire—techniques like sponging, stenciling, and layering colors to give depth and dimension to a room or wall. We had a client who had three children and had just gone through a divorce. She hired us to make over her bedroom in three shades of purple.

When we had finished and re-assembled the room, we walked her—with her eyes closed—to the doorway. When she opened her eyes, she began almost immediately to cry, as did we. For years, her ex-husband had insisted on neutral colors, so everything was either off-white or gray. As she stood in the doorway of her own bedroom done her way, her "happy" hormones took over and melted away some of the stress of her divorce. And that effect would be repeated every time she walked into her bedroom.

When people fill their minds and their days with never-ending to-do lists, they tend to be swamped with stress and stress hormones that kick their brains into constant survival mode.

By finding periods of time each day to be happy, and by implementing surroundings that put a sincere smile on your face, you give happy hormones a chance to offset stress hormones. A happy brain functions more efficiently, sleeps better, stimulates immune function and bone regeneration, plus many more healthy responses.

Simple Solutions:

- Consume enough water. Start with one to two quarts per day. That's the equivalent of four to eight cups of clean, preferably filtered water.

- Good nutrition, even in snack foods. (More on this in the next chapter.)

- Adequate sleep. My suggestion is six to eight hours per night. Quality sleep is a major issue for many people, and there are healthy choices for sleep aids. One way to improve sleep habits is to lower your stimulation in the evening—turn off the television earlier, do not watch late-night news, do not work or surf the internet. (Hopefully, you're not reading this too late at night—unless you find it soothing or even a bit boring. If so, then congrats and sweet dreams!)

- Take a short siesta during the day. Even ten minutes of undisturbed rest can be invaluable to healthy brain recuperation. Undisturbed means no email, Facebook, or phone calls. Try just sitting in the sunshine and fresh air with eyes closed to rest the brain from its usual state of stimulation.

- Organize your work area, be it your desk, office space, or even stacks of papers that have piled up. Cluttered spaces tend to accentuate the things you should be getting to or tasks that have been completed but are still clogging an area on your desk.

- Brain exercises. There are mental exercises specifically designed to enhance memory, and many can be found on the internet.

7

Healthy Snacking and Weight Control

CAUTION WITH THAT VENDING MACHINE

We cannot solve problems by using the same kind of thinking we used when we created them.

—Albert Einstein

The importance of healthy eating to achieving your best performance cannot be stressed enough. After all, NASA did not put regular unleaded fuel in the space shuttles. It may seem a stretch to compare our brains and bodies to spacecraft headed for orbit, but there is room for this comparison. The shuttle needed an elaborate computer system to oversee and maintain all of its systems. All the technology that enabled the shuttle to operate can be likened to our body and brain. Most of the computer workings of the shuttle are at the head of the spacecraft, the cockpit, just as our heads are atop our bodies.

As there are thousands of people required to run a space mission, our bodies have a number of systems working together to operate our "shuttle." At the helm is the brain, and the fuel for the brain determines how well it operates. This may sound simplistic, and it is! But there is still a lot that goes into the process.

Our brain and body require a certain amount of nutrients to adequately fuel the many thousands of functions they perform daily. If those nutrient needs are not met, we literally are in a state of hunger, no matter how many calories have been consumed. And hungry brains are not happy brains.

The snacks and meals you choose can make a significant difference in how you feel at the end of the day, how well your brain functions throughout the day, and what your waistline tells you at the end of the week or month. This concept has been illustrated over and over with humans in all stages of life and development.

A dear friend's daughter attended a public school that was part of an experiment conducted with fourth through sixth graders. For a month, the choices offered in the cafeteria were healthy—salads and wholesome entrees with quality side dishes. Although some students initially rebelled at the change in the menu (no pizza, no hot dogs, no french fries, no mac and cheese), they came around, as there were no alternatives.

Over the course of the month, teachers, administrators, and even the students themselves noted a marked change in attitudes and behaviors. There were fewer class outbursts, but an increase in class participation. That participation was improved by students' calmer behavior and increased ability to focus on lessons and instructions. And this was only one month of diet change, with no other differing variables. Due to budget restrictions, the experiment had to conclude, but imagine the benefits if it were extended, or even made permanent?

When my sister and I were teenagers, the reality of our hard-working, single-mom-led household was that we spent many an evening in front of the TV with a frozen dinner or fast food. That dynamic is even more prevalent today, as more parents work multiple jobs and there are more single-parent households.

In my early twenties, I signed up for a nutrition class a friend told me about at the local community college. The focus was vegetarianism and whole food nutrition, and I took to the information like a duck to water. That was thirty years ago, and I still use things I learned in that class as guideposts for food choices today.

In naturopathic medicine, we often say that a treatment should be implemented for three months to give it time to change body patterns. Can you imagine applying the lessons learned at that public school to our workforce for a three-month period? Making healthier choices about meals and snacks can have an incredible impact not only on your health, but also on your productivity at work and your ability to focus on detail-oriented tasks.

Nutritionists classify food according to nutrient density. Foods with empty calories have a high calorie count but little nutritional benefit. Nutrient-dense options have far more beneficial substances in a comparable amount of food. For example, a typical can of soda contains seven to fourteen teaspoons of sugar and almost no vitamins or minerals. A big glass of milk or nut milk; i.e., almond, coconut, etc., has protein, vitamin A, vitamin C, thiamin, riboflavin, and niacin, plus minerals, calcium, and iron. There's a huge difference in nutritional value between those two twelve-ounce amounts of liquid.

Other examples of low- to high-nutrient density comparisons include: ketchup vs. salsa, candy bars vs. high-quality protein bars, potato chips vs. trail mix. A typical serving size of chips is about an ounce, or approximately eleven chips, which contains about 140–188 calories, with 60%–64% of the calories coming from fat. Over the course of a year, these calories can lead to ten to twenty pounds gained. So think about replacing that handful of chips with a measured amount of trail mix or—even better—a bowl of grapes or an apple.

Whole grain crackers are a great salty crunch with a lower calorie count. For more crunch factor, try celery, carrots, or even sweet red peppers with a side of salsa, hummus, or bean dip. Healthy snacks in an office setting can be more of a challenge, but suggesting and bringing healthier alternatives often is a better strategy than eliminating someone's favorite snack. Co-workers can collaborate to make sure that there is something available for everyone.

In today's market, there are healthier versions of just about any snack food; you just have to look a little harder until you find them.

The Gut-Brain Connection

In human anatomy, there are two routes of exposing our inner world to the influences of the outer world. One is our breath, which is hopefully occurring on a regular basis, and the other is the food we eat. In a book that is prominent on my reference shelf, *The Second Brain: Your Gut Has a Mind of its Own*, Dr. Michael D. Gershon shows the direct connection between our gut and our brain. By explaining how intimately these two organs relate to each other, Gershon provides evidence that proves how the health of our gut has a significant impact on the health of our brain.

There is a direct link between the hormone serotonin, also known as the happy hormone, and a healthy small intestine. In the past decade or so, research has confirmed that the majority of serotonin is produced by the small intestine, and that the health of our gastrointestinal tract dictates the amount of hormone produced. That makes it even more important to fuel our bodies properly!

Having the ability to focus in our lives, jobs, or any other area of interest, for that matter, starts with what we eat on a daily basis. There are many things in life that we have little control over, but we can control what we eat and how much we eat every day.

By making healthier and tastier food choices, you can literally change your mood, physical well-being, and the outcome of your day.

The human brain runs almost entirely on blood sugar, otherwise known as blood glucose. Almost all sugars are made up of part glucose and some other molecules. In order for our brain to get its needed fuel and run efficiently, it must get a regular supply of this blood glucose. It has been proven that a slow, steady supply of blood sugar keeps our brain happier than a massive dose followed by a period of low levels, also known as hypoglycemia.

Complex carbohydrates—foods with sugars and fiber—are digested in a manner that produces this time-release supply of blood sugar. Think about an apple, peel and all. Simple carbohydrates, such as apple juice, are more easily absorbed and cause quicker blood-sugar spikes. You can apply this strategy to all manner of snacks and beverages—the more fiber, proteins, and healthy fats, the more stable the production of blood sugar.

Another important element is the difference between whole fruit and dehydrated fruit. The dehydrated fruit contains almost all the healthy aspects of the original fruit, but its lack of water (food volume) makes it much easier to overeat. Eating one or two mini-size boxes of raisins isn't too hard; there can be about thirty raisins in one box. But try eating thirty grapes with their full water content. After eating that many grapes, you're going to have a greater feeling of fullness than after the mini box of raisins, not to mention your thirst will also have been satisfied.

Maintaining balanced blood sugars is essential on several levels—brain function and clarity, emotional stability, lowered stress on adrenal glands, and a more equalized energy level throughout the day. Low blood sugar is interpreted by our body and brain as stress, and the adrenal glands are intimately involved in managing it.

Mismanagement of blood sugar produces low energy levels, which we often then try to ameliorate with caffeine. But caffeine, ingested into an empty digestive system, has a similar effect on the adrenal glands as a minor jolt of electricity! This is not to say that a cup of coffee is a bad thing, but moderation and timing are crucial to keeping that cup of joe from kicking your body into stressful fight-or-flight mode.

Don't drink coffee on an empty stomach, and choose your additives carefully. Plant-based Stevia adds sweetness without spiking blood sugar or calorie intake. A teaspoon of unpasteurized honey is a better choice than cane sugar, and a splash of coconut- or almond-milk creamer mixes well in coffee without adding to its acidity. (You might also consider coffee alternatives such as black tea or chai.)

It's conventional wisdom that caffeine has a stimulating effect on brain function, sharpness, and alertness. But with access to new technologies, brain activity is easier to monitor today. This monitoring has shown that caffeine actually binds to a receptor site in the brain that's responsible for relaxation—that area of the brain allows you to relax and get calm. Caffeine's binding to this receptor site interferes with that process, meaning you stay stimulated or more awake.

These receptor sites that caffeine can bind to are not just in the brain. They're throughout the body—heart, lungs, etc. This is why most people notice their heart rate speeds up after drinking coffee, or they get jittery and feel more alert. As with influxes of sugar and simple carbohydrates, influxes of caffeine lead to "crashes." Once the body clears caffeine from those binding sites, people feel more tired than before, prompting them to reach for another cup of coffee or caffeine-laden energy drink to keep going.

I don't want to label coffee as the only culprit in our energy deficit; we have busier lives and are sleeping less than many generations before us. But in many cases when I directed my patients to eliminate coffee for a week, they would report back that their energy levels improved and they felt more alert during the day.

Additionally, the acidity in coffee and other foods and beverages has earned its place in causing other symptoms for many people. Common complaints are GERD (gastroesophageal reflux disease), acid reflux, heartburn, and a burning or gnawing sensation in the stomach, just to mention a few. As with most symptoms, these are a sign of something else going on in your body. Increased acidity—which is a lowered pH of the blood—leads to a host of other health issues.

Stress, regardless of its cause, can contribute to increased acidity. As with anything, acidity is all a matter of degree. When acid levels rise in the blood, some biochemical pathway functions are negatively affected. An example of this would be digestion. Acid is required to digest proteins, but too much acid can interfere with the digestion of other food groups, such as carbohydrates and fats. This causes fat-soluble vitamins, such as vitamin A, to not be absorbed well, which eventually leads to a deficiency of those vitamins.

Sugary foods and beverages are referred to as acidifying foods, meaning they cause an increase in the amount of how much acid is produced to digest them. Alkalizing foods and beverages have the opposite effect. Almost all fruits and vegetables, herbal teas, and certain nuts, seeds, and grains fall into this category. When fruits or veggies are eaten, blood pH becomes more alkaline, and a more alkaline pH helps create balance in stress-filled lives.

To clarify, stress, whether unhealthy or healthy, can be damaging to our overall well-being. The good news is that one avenue toward controlling our stress levels is to control what we eat and drink through the course of a day. By choosing healthier versions of foods, drinks, and snacks, we can literally shift our blood acid or pH levels.

Quantity or Quality

Prioritizing quantity over quality, in my opinion, is part of the reason we have such an obesity epidemic in this country. When looking at why many people overeat, I believe it has to do with the poor quality of many popular and inexpensive food options.

There is also an element of overly busy lives and fast-food convenience, which in the long run is not so convenient. One of the mottos in our clinic was "everything in moderation" (unless dealing with a health issue). I believe in the 80%/20% rule, where eating well and taking care of yourself 80% of the time will compensate for the 20% that you may not be taking such good care of yourself.

Options, Not Deprivation

I have learned over the years, when asking patients to change their diet, that it is extremely important to not just take a food item or food group away, but to replace it with a healthier version that tastes good. By incorporating this replacement idea, my patients rarely feel deprived, and the benefits prove worth the effort.

Exploring options for snack foods, several considerations come to mind. Convenience, ease of access, taste, and cost seem to rank at the top of the list. By considering convenience first, you should also include how that snack food is going to affect your mood, productivity, and general feeling of well-being. An example of a healthy choice would be reaching for a quality energy bar instead of a candy bar. Eating snacks that are high in sugar but not protein and fat, like candy bars, will result in a rapid blood sugar spike that will end in an energy-level crash.

Today, there are many types of snack bars available at a reasonable cost, and planning for them to become a regular snack food would mean you could buy in bulk to save money and time. A key component when choosing an energy bar is the ratio of carbohydrate (50%) to protein (20%) and fat (30%)—hopefully healthy fat.

Another problem associated with a poor choice in snack foods, especially candy or sugary snacks, is how excess sugar is converted into triglycerides, a type of fat stored in your body. Without going into a full nutrition class here, this is a major reason as to why waistlines increase at the end of the year even though people don't think they've eaten more than usual. The problem isn't necessarily with the amount of calories consumed, but the type of calories and a lack of physical activity.

Throughout my years in private practice and nutritional counseling, I have witnessed amazing changes in my patients when even moderate alterations have been made to their dietary habits. In several instances, when replacing sugary foods and drinks such as sodas, they would report back with surprise as to how their energy levels had improved and stayed more balanced throughout the day. In this case, we are going to bridge energy levels with thinking processes and stability of mood. Very often, my patients would comment on how they couldn't believe the difference in their mood swings, or lack thereof, just from making better food and snack choices.

Making a switch in my diet some thirty years ago has made a huge difference in my health today. When everyone around me is getting sick, either in the fall or winter with a cold or the flu, I may get a little something, but nothing compared with those around me. I suffered from allergies as a child, but that all changed when I committed myself to eating differently. Even today, when there is an occasional splurge, like pizza, there is usually a price to pay.

Using pizza as an example, in teaching cooking classes, I became aware of gluten-free pizza dough that tasted just fine with enough doctoring. In fact, in the class, the students couldn't tell the difference in the crust because of the toppings I included and the wonderful sauce I used. Luckily, I am aware of numerous ways to integrate alternatives, so there is never a reason to do without a particular food. I just buy or make a healthier version.

Simple Solutions:

- A bowl of grapes, preferably organic (to avoid pesticide and other spray residues).

- Trail mix, but in measured amounts. Otherwise it is too easy to just keep eating this snack, and you'll have consumed 300–400 calories before you know it.

- One to two tablespoons of nut butter (almond, peanut, or other) and celery, apple, crackers, a banana. (I understand Elvis liked peanut butter and banana sandwiches.)

- An apple with some cheese.

- Carrots (even steamed or sautéed). This can satisfy a crunch and calorie need.

- Any type of vegetable, such as kale chips, zucchini chips, red peppers, or edamame.

- Some form of dip—hummus, black bean, salsa—and steamed broccoli or leftover grilled vegetables.

- Two or three small pieces of fruit. Cut up melons make for a wonderful pick-me-up.

- Unsweetened herbal tea (add your own sweetener) or chai. Quality fruit juice, preferably diluted with water or seltzer to reduce calorie and sugar intake.

- Did I mention clean, filtered water? Adding a squeeze of lemon juice or apple cider vinegar (I know this may sound a bit strange, but it works) balances what I call stress-induced acidity in the body.

CONCLUSION

Lord, give us this day our daily miracle and forgive us if we don't recognize it.

> *The best six doctors anywhere,*
> *and no one can deny it,*
> *are sunshine, water, rest, and air,*
> *exercise and diet.*
> *These six will gladly you attend,*
> *if only you are willing.*
> *Your mind they'll ease,*
> *your will they'll mend,*
> *and charge you not a shilling.*
>
> —*Wayne Fields*

USEFUL LINKS

1. https://www.health.harvard.edu/diseases-and-conditions/ glycemic-index-and-glycemic-load-for-100-foods

2. http://www.infoplease.com/ipa/A0931441.html

3. http://www.governing.com/blogs/view/gov-us-youth-spend-more-time-on-computers-less-in-front-of-tv.html

4. http://www.clotcare.com/faq_graduatedcompressionstock-ings.aspx

5. http://www.huffingtonpost.com/2012/11/10/memory-loss-meds-to-blame_n_2094842.html

6. http://www.ncbi.nlm.nih.gov/pmc/articles/PMC2077351/ (serotonin levels, how to raise without drugs)

7. http://www.integrativepsychiatry.net/serotonin.html (treatments and foods to raise serotonin)

8. http://www.chai-tea.org/whatisit.html

9. http://faculty.washington.edu/chudler/caff.html

10. https://www.mayoclinic.org/healthy-lifestyle/fitness/multi-media/stretching/sls-20076840 (stretching videos)

REFERENCES

Introduction

Grohol, J. (2020, July 06). Depression: Symptoms, Types & Treatments. Retrieved October 27, 2020, from https://psychcentral.com/depression/

Psychologist, J. (2020, January 16). Does Social Media Cause Depression? Retrieved October 27, 2020, from https://www.scientificamerican.com/article/does-social-media-cause-depression/

Chapter 1

Households with Computers, 1998 – 2010. (n.d.). Retrieved October 27, 2020, from http://www.infoplease.com/ipa/A0931441.html

U.S. Youth Spend More Time on Computers, Less in Front of TV. Retrieved October 27, 2020, from http://www.governing.com/blogs/view/gov-us-youth-spend-more-time-on-computers-less-in-front-of-tv.html

Elroy Boers, P. (2019, September 01). Association of Screen Time and Depression in Adolescence. Retrieved October 27, 2020, from https://jamanetwork.com/journals/jamapediatrics/article-abstract/2737909?guestAccessKey=f3fe2ed6-1fb3-44cc-a9a8-a38bd0463942

Chapter 2

Clement, J. (2020, January 07). Number of internet users worldwide. Retrieved October 27, 2020, from https://www.statista.com/statistics/273018/number-of-internet-users-worldwide/

Eye strain. (n.d.). Retrieved October 27, 2020, from https://www.the-londonclinic.co.uk/conditions/eye-strain

Charles Patrick Davis, M. (2016, September 08). Sick Building Syndrome Symptoms & Prevention. Retrieved October 27, 2020, from http://www.medicinenet.com/sick_building_syndrome/article.htm

Publishing, H. (n.d.). Blue light has a dark side. Retrieved October 27, 2020, from https://www.health.harvard.edu/staying-healthy/blue-light-has-a-dark-side

Arjmandi, N., Mortazavi, G., Zarei, S., Faraz, M., & Mortazavi, S. (2018, December 1). Can Light Emitted from Smartphone Screens and Taking Selfies Cause Premature Aging and Wrinkles? Retrieved October 27, 2020, from https://www.ncbi.nlm.nih.gov/pmc/articles/PMC6280109/

Ryan, C. L., & U.S. Census Bureau,. (2018). *Computer and internet use in the United States: 2016.*

Eyestrain. (2020, August 28). Retrieved October 27, 2020, from https://www.mayoclinic.org/diseases-conditions/eyestrain/diagnosis-treatment/drc-20372403

Publishing, H. (n.d.). Blue light has a dark side. Retrieved October 27, 2020, from https://www.health.harvard.edu/staying-healthy/blue-light-has-a-dark-side

Chapter 3

George Ansstas, M. (2019, November 09). Vitamin A Deficiency. Retrieved October 27, 2020, from http://emedicine.medscape.com/article/126004-overview

Skin Turgor. (n.d.). Retrieved October 27, 2020, from https://www.sciencedirect.com/topics/biochemistry-genetics-and-molecular-biology/skin-turgor

Chapter 5

Deep vein thrombosis (DVT). (2018, March 06). Retrieved October 27, 2020, from https://www.mayoclinic.org/diseases-conditions/deep-vein-thrombosis/symptoms-causes/syc-20352557

Chapter 6

How the Fight-or-Flight response explains stress. (n.d.). How Fight-or-flight Instincts Impact On Your Stress Levels. Retrieved October 27, 2020, from https://www.psychologistworld.com/stress/fight-or-flight-response

Vitamin D. (2020, October 19). Retrieved October 27, 2020, from https://www.hsph.harvard.edu/nutritionsource/vitamin-d/

Chapter 7

How Can I Eat More Nutrient-Dense Foods? (n.d.). Retrieved October 27, 2020, from https://www.heart.org/en/healthy-living/healthy-eating/eat-smart/nutrition-basics/how-can-i-eat-more-nutrient-dense-foods

The Simplified Guide to the Gut-Brain Axis - How the Gut Talks to the Brain. (n.d.). Retrieved October 27, 2020, from https://psychscenehub.com/psychinsights/the-simplified-guide-to-the-gut-brain-axis/

Images

Fig 1. Sick Building https://livepureinc.com/wp-content/uploads/2018/04/sick-house-syndrome-toxins.jpg

Fig 2. Anatomy of Sitting https://www.bigstockphoto.com/image-215007073/stock-vector-the-lumbar-region-is-sometimes-referred-to-as-the-lower-spine-or-as-an-area-of-the-back-in-its-proximity

Fig 3. Bowling Ball Created by Lisa Dixon for Vital Health Publishing.

Fig 4. Head position https://www.bigstockphoto.com/image-10423328/stock-photo-boy-with-laptop

Fig 5. Head tilt https://www.bigstockphoto.com/image-195611095/stock-vector-sport-exercises-for-office-office-yoga-for-tired-employees-with-chair-and-table-neck-stretching

Fig 6. Neck stretch https://musculoskeletalkey.com/neck-assessment/

Fig 7. Neck flexion. https://tinyurl.com/y4djbcve

Fig 8. Shoulder stretch Image: Cancer Research UK / Wikimedia Commons

Fig 9. Shoulder roll Image: Cancer Research UK / Wikimedia Commons

Fig 10. CTS https://www.bigstockphoto.com/image-24280364/stock-vector-transverse-carpal-ligament

Fig 11. Ergonomic wrists https://www.bigstockphoto.com/image-300786619/stock-vector-carpal-tunnel-syndrome-infographic%2C-health-concept-%0Aflat-design-illustration-businessman-businessm

Fig 12. Wrist flexion https://www.bigstockphoto.com/image-300786619/stock-vector-carpal-tunnel-syndrome-infographic%2C-health-concept-%0Aflat-design-illustration-businessman-businessm

Fig 13. Wrist extension https://www.bigstockphoto.com/image-300786619/stock-vector-carpal-tunnel-syndrome-infographic%2C-health-concept-%0Aflat-design-illustration-businessman-businessm

Fig 14. Finger exercises https://www.bigstockphoto.com/image-300786619/stock-vector-carpal-tunnel-syndrome-infographic%2C-health-concept-%0Aflat-design-illustration-businessman-businessm

Fig 15. DVT https://www.nycsurgical.net/assets/08-09-11-dvt-jpg040611fa_revised.jpg

Fig 16. Leg and calf https://www.bigstockphoto.com/image-190943008/stock-vector-sport-exercises-for-office-office-yoga-for-tired-employees-with-chair-and-table-legs-workout

Fig 17. Foot roller https://tinyurl.com/y6eerh8z

Fig 18. Mental overload https://tinyurl.com/y6fewn86

About the Author

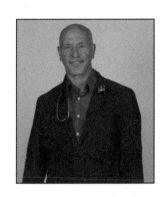

Mitchell A. Kershner, ND
Naturopathic Doctor
Drmitchellkershner.com
info@drmitchellnd.com

Mitchell Kershner, ND, is a naturopathic doctor who has been in the health field for more than thirty-two years. His studies began in the field of nutrition at Miami Dade Community College in 1985. He continued his studies in personal fitness and later became a trainer at several local gyms, spas, and health clubs.

After doing extensive work in nutrition and going on to receive a license for massage therapy in 1989, he thought to himself, "There must be a profession that combines these fields of health care along with my interest in exercise." This thought led him to seek and find naturopathic medicine. Upon completing his prerequisites at Florida International University, he moved to Portland, Oregon, to study naturopathic medicine at the National College of Naturopathic Medicine.

Upon graduation in 1996, he relocated to Taos, New Mexico, and opened his private practice. Three years into practice, he started teaching at the University of New Mexico in the nursing program biology/science department. Kershner started teaching clinical nutrition at the undergraduate level and went on to teach anatomy and physiology. He also taught exercise physiology to the massage program students.

During his stay in northern New Mexico, Kershner served as a medical crew member on the Taos Search and Rescue team.

Aging family and a desire to pursue more education in the culinary world brought Kershner back to South Florida, where he attended culinary school and received a diploma equivalent in culinary arts from the International Culinary School at the Art Institutes in Fort Lauderdale. In November 2011, he started *Healthy Chef Doctor*, a company dedicated to health education through guest lecturing, simple and healthy cooking demonstrations, private events, and home parties.

His creation of *Working from Home: Mastering the Art of Sitting at Your Computer* is the culmination of his work in optimal body posture and function while incorporating the naturopathic medicine approach. It is his offering to all those who sit at a computer for work or school to help prevent computer related conditions. As the saying goes, "An ounce of prevention is worth more than a pound of cure."